DATE DUE

unpr

fo

eavitt

retary

JUL   2000

#23

THE

BIRD
FLU

PREPAREDNESS PLANNER

What it is.
How it spreads.
What you can do.

GRATTAN WOODSON, M.D.
EDITED BY DAVID JODREY, PH.D.

Health Communications, Inc.
Deerfield Beach, Florida

www.bcibooks.com

This book is not intended to be a substitute for the advice and/or medical care of the reader's physician, nor is it meant to dissuade the reader from the advice of his or her physician. The reader should consult with a physician in all matters related to his or her health.

©2005 Grattan Woodson
ISBN 0-7573-0498-2

Publisher: Health Communications, Inc.
          3201 S.W. 15th Street
          Deerfield Beach, FL 33442-8190

Cover design by Larissa Hise Henoch
Inside book design by Dawn Von Strolley Grove

Contents

Introduction

Chances are, if you've opened a newspaper or turned on the news in 2005, you might be worried, perhaps even a little panicked, about the avian flu or bird flu—and with good reason. What many people around the world dismissed as a minor headline in the International section of their newspaper seemed to mushroom overnight into a global health crisis.

And a crisis it is. Right now, scientists, physicians and government officials around the world are waging war against H5N1, a super strain of one of humankind's oldest and most persistent pathogens—the influenza virus. But this is no ordinary flu virus: This new strain is highly lethal, with a death rate of fifty percent, 80 times the normal flu, with the potential to kill hundreds of millions given the right conditions. Those conditions are in place right now, according to the World Health Organization and the U.S. Centers for Disease Control and Prevention, not alarmist groups and extremists.

If not contained, the avian flu has the potential to spread like wildfire, much like the Spanish Flu of 1918 which killed 50 million worldwide. If you find it difficult to imagine what a pandemic flu would mean to you in the United States, picture the aftermath of Hurricane Katrina, and then multiply it by every state (and then, every continent). If pandemic flu hit North America, it would decimate every state, leaving death, destruction and chaos in its wake; and, unlike during a hurricane, you couldn't ride out its wrath hunkered down in your closet for a few hours, because a pandemic flu would last many months—perhaps a year or more.

What happened in New Orleans during and after Hurricane Katrina has shown us two things: Sometimes we are unlucky enough to have the "worst case" come true; and, we as a society are woefully unprepared for it.

And while some nay-sayers may roll their eyes, the question is not *if* a pandemic will happen, but when. The questions we need to ask ourselves are "Would I be ready?" "Do I have what it takes to survive?"

I wrote this preparedness manual for my patients. I wrote it to inform them about this growing health threat and to provide them with practical guidance on how they and their families can survive. The question is not whether we will have another pandemic: It is certain that we will. What is not known is whether it will be a major one like the 1918 flu which killed 50 million people worldwide, or a "minor" one like the 1957 flu pandemic which killed more than 1 million people. My advice: Prepare for the worst and hope for the best. This manual will show you how.

How to Use This Book

In this book I will give you the facts, not fiction; science, not scare tactics. The first few sections will give you background information about the influenza virus, with special attention on the 1918 Spanish Flu, the last major pandemic.

The second half of the book gives you practical suggestions and preparedness plans you should put in place now given the extremely disruptive effect a major pandemic would have on society and essential services. You'll learn some essential foods, medicines and supplies you should have in your home, what decisions you and your loved ones need to make now in the event the unthinkable happens, as well as medical advice for both laypeople and medical professionals who find themselves caring for those stricken with the avian flu.

As the world saw during Hurricane Katrina, many people suffered because they trusted their care to others. The reality is, in most crisis situations, it's the people who are prepared, not panicked, who survive. In this book I will give you the information you need to prepare.

H5N1: The Next Pandemic?

A highly virulent and deadly new influenza virus strain is emerging in Southeast Asia that is of great concern to health administrators and infectious disease specialists. The new virus is called H5N1 avian influenza virus type A. Many infectious disease experts think we are on the verge of a major worldwide influenza pandemic of similar severity to the 1918 Spanish Flu.

What Is a Pandemic?

An epidemic is defined as an infectious illness that spreads so quickly that the number of new cases rises in an exponential manner rather than just increasing linearly. This means that the number of new cases doesn't just go up by ones or twos each day, but doubles every few days. A pandemic is an outbreak of disease that affects every continent rather than just one geographic area.

One of the most important reasons for influenza's success in spreading epidemics is its *infectivity,* or how easily it is transmitted from one person to another. Infectious agents that can cause illness after a small exposure are more contagious than ones that require a larger exposure. Infectivity is increased when infection can be passed between people without any direct contact.

The most common way for flu to be transmitted is by breathing contaminated air. It can also be transmitted by direct contact with an infected person, shaking a hand or touching something that the sick person previously touched. Under the right conditions, flu can remain infectious for days outside of the human body, living on surfaces like counter tops or doorknobs.

The virus can only infect someone if that person is susceptible or vulnerable to it. Unfortunately, virtually 100 percent of the human population is susceptible to a new strain of virus, like avian flu, because we don't have any immunity to it.

Influenza causes pandemics because it scores so highly in all these causes of infectivity. These characteristics of influenza help explain why this organism can quickly spread from one region of the globe to another.

During flu pandemics, a higher than usual percentage of the population becomes infected and more people die than during the usual annual flu season. Pandemics occur because a new influenza virus makes its way from birds or swine to humans, resulting in a strain for which we have very little immunity.

Major and Minor Pandemics

There are major pandemics and minor ones. Minor ones are more common and much less severe than major ones, but still a lot worse than routine flu outbreaks we experience each winter. All pandemics infect many times more people than happens with the seasonal flu but during major pandemics, like the Spanish Flu

Mortality Rate from Influenza in the United States
(Per 100,000 People)

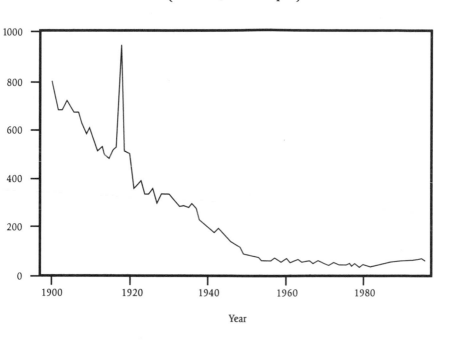

Year

Note the spike in deaths during the 1918-1919 Spanish Flu epidemic.

Source: Center for Disease Control (CDC)

of 1918, the death rates soar into the tens of millions or even higher.

On average there are two minor pandemics for every one major pandemic. The minor pandemics are associated with lower clinical attack and case fatality rates than in major pandemics. For instance, the 1957 pandemic was associated with three times as many deaths than seen for seasonal flu but during the 1968 flu pandemic, there were only a few more deaths than would be expected. It has now been thirty-seven years since the last flu pandemic, which suggests we may be due for another one soon.

Pandemic Death Tolls

During the 1918-1919 pandemic, five to ten times as many people as usual became severely ill with flu, and many millions died from their infection. The percentage of the population that becomes ill with flu symptoms is known as the *clinical attack rate.* The medical term for the percentage of people who become ill and die is the *case fatality rate.* During the usual winter flu season, the case fatality rate hovers around 0.2 percent to 0.35 percent. During minor pandemics, this rate increases up to 3 to 4 times; during a major pandemic the rate increases by 10 to 50 times!

Pandemics Can Be Predicted

One of the things that surprises many people is that influenza pandemics are regular events with an almost predictable periodicity of three per century. In fact, over the last four hundred years there have been twelve recorded flu pandemics. Every hundred years or so, a major pandemic occurs that dwarfs everything else by comparison.

Most flu experts predict that it is only a matter of time before the bird flu virus mutates to become transmissible between people, so that is not the burning question. The question is: how soon?

According to the World Health Organization guidelines for pandemics, as of September 2005 we are in Phase 3. This places us in the Pandemic Alert Period, just one step away from human-to-human spread that will be followed by a worldwide pandemic. Even during the relatively primitive travel conditions existing in 1918, it took only six weeks for epidemic influenza to spread from the United States to Europe and Africa. Imagine how fast the next pandemic virus will move across the globe given the many thousands of passengers traveling internationally by air every day. Taking this into account, the British Government's Health Protection Agency predicts in their Influenza Pandemic Contingency Plan that once the first case of pandemic flu reaches Hong Kong it will take only two to weeks to arrive in the United Kingdom.

My estimate is that when the avian flu crosses over to humans, there is a one in three chance of a major pandemic and a two out of three chance of a minor one. The most likely time for this to happen in the Northern Hemisphere is during the annual flu season from December 2005 through March 2006. This estimate is based on several factors. Most virologists agree that for H5N1 to achieve efficient human-to-human transmission it will require more human flu RNA; the time when this is most likely to happen is during the annual flu season which runs from December through March. The next most likely time would be December 2006 through April 2007.

WHO Pandemic Phases

INTERPANDEMIC PERIOD

Phase 1. No new influenza virus subtypes detected in humans although there are some endemic in animals that have infected humans.

Phase 2. No new influenza virus sub-types detected in humans, but a circulating animal sub-type poses a substantial risk to human health.

PANDEMIC ALERT PERIOD

Phase 3. Human infection(s) confirmed with new sub-type but no or only minimal human-to-human spread among close contacts.

Phase 4. Small clusters with limited human-to-human transmission but spread is highly localized, suggesting that the virus is not well adapted to humans.

Phase 5. Larger clusters but human-to-human spread still localized, suggesting that the virus is becoming increasingly better adapted to humans, but may not yet be fully transmissible (substantial pandemic risk).

PANDEMIC PERIOD

Phase 6. Pandemic: increased and sustained transmission in general population.

Source: The WHO http://www.who.int/csr/resources/publications/influenza/WHO_CDS_CSR_GIP_2005_5.pdf

Influenza pandemics occur in waves. The 1918 Spanish Flu (H1N1) was associated with three waves, while the 1957 Asian Flu (H2N2) and 1968 Hong Kong Flu (H3N2) had two distinct waves each. The reason for this wave behavior is not known, but some speculate it's due to a change in the season of the year. The timing of a wave may also be related to a genetic change or mutation in the new strain of influenza virus. In past pandemics, the time between two waves was three to nine months. One point to keep in mind about pandemic waves is that the second wave can be much more severe than the first or third wave of the series. During the 1918 pandemic, the deadly second wave was responsible for more than 90 percent of the deaths for the entire pandemic.

While the typical flu season predictably occurs from November through March, during pandemics, flu can vary from this script. The first wave of the 1918 flu spanned January through March. That flu was very severe by usual standards but the second wave, beginning six months later in September, was the most fatal. The third wave occurred during the following winter/spring and was the mildest of all. Pandemics end, not because of a miracle cure or a magic-bullet vaccine, but simply because all or most susceptible persons within the population have contracted the infection and developed immunity to it, or they died.

Pandemics Strike the Healthiest, Too

During pandemics, a major difference compared with seasonal flu is that there is a high death rate among healthy twenty- to thirty-year-old adults. This is in contrast with the seasonal flu that strikes the very old, the young, and the infirm the hardest. Of course, the usual victims of seasonal flu are not spared during pandemics. On the contrary, death rates are much higher for every age and risk group during pandemics compared with seasonal flu. The point here is that the twenty-to-thirty- year-old group, usually immune to the ravages of seasonal flu, experiences very high death rates. Ironically, one possible explanation for this pandemic observation may relate to the increased health and vigor of this group's immune system.

What Makes the
Avian Flu So Fearsome?

A vian influenza H5N1 is so troubling to the medical community because of its stunning killing ability, a statistic known as the *lethality* of the disease. The 1918 flu, like most pandemics, infected 40 to 50 percent of the world's population or approximately 640 million people. If we assume that approximately 50 million people died during the 1918 influenza pandemic this is a case fatality rate of about 12.5 percent of those infected. What is so worrisome to the influenza experts at the U.S. CDC and WHO is the case fatality rate for humans infected with the avian flu is approximately 50 percent. While this number may overstate the true lethality to an extent, as there may well be a number of milder cases who have not come to the attention of the health authorities, nevertheless, these fatalities show how deadly the virus can be.

Right now, the virus is confined mostly to birds, but has adapted to tigers and pigs. Almost all of the humans infected have had contact with infected birds during processing, cooking, eating, caring for them, or visiting the zoo. However, experts are paying close attention for any sign that H5N1 avian influenza has become more efficient in person-to-person spread, either from mutation or from swapping genes with another flu variety in an infected person or animal. If this event occurs, the new viral offspring would gain the ability to spread directly from person to person. This development would signal the beginning of the pandemic.

Human-to-Human Transmission

What was believed to be the first documented case of person-to-person transmission of avian flu in Thailand in 2004 was reported in the *New England Journal of Medicine.*[1] That strain did not spread further in people. However, as this is being written, in early fall 2005, a number of troubling cases of family clusters are being reported in Indonesia. Dr. Henry Niman, a virologist, discusses these cases on his Web site, *www.recominomics.com*, pointing out that the World Health Organization's diagnostic criteria for bird flu were not met by many of the patients apparently ill with the disease because of the timing of test specimen collection. These technical errors resulted in many instances of patients who didn't meet the fourfold increase in antibody levels to bird flu, or some who didn't have the bird flu virus in their nose and throat at the time the testing for RNA was conducted. These technical difficulties prevented the government from confirming bird flu despite the impressions of physicians and scientists that almost all were certainly infected with the virus. This is Dr. Niman's conclusion, and I think he's correct.

How Lethal Will It Be?

If and when a bird flu virus that spreads well between people emerges, we cannot be certain how lethal this new virus will be. It is not likely to be as lethal as native H5N1 avian flu has been to the people who have caught it from birds, but will probably be a lot worse than routine seasonal flu. While no one can predict this in advance, history and computer models predict that there is one in three chance that it would have a worldwide clinical attack rate of 35 to 50 percent and a case fatality rate of 3 to 10 percent of the population. If this proves to be the case, the effect on humanity and society will be traumatic in ways thought impossible today in light of advances in technology and medicine.

According to Michael Osterholm, Ph.D.,[2] in the *New England Journal of Medicine,* the most likely scenario if we have a major pandemic, is for an event that approximates the death toll seen during 1918 Spanish Flu.[3] On the other hand, if reassortment of H5N1 avian flu with human influenza results in a pandemic of the minor variety this would not represent a dire threat to humanity or lead to any significant disruption in our social or economic life.

Right now, we're relying on probabilities and expert estimates that suggest there is a one in three chance the next pandemic will be of the major variety. Government in the U.S. and Europe tend to focus on the hoped-for two in three chance that the next pandemic will be of the minor variety.[4,5] No doubt these sanguine estimates are affected by government policies, politics and fears of upsetting the public.

These influences may explain why the government prediction for the clinical attack rate is at the low end for pandemics, and why the predicted case fatality rates are the same as those seen during seasonal influenza. Higher and more realistic morbidity and mortality estimates are beginning to emerge in the press and in television and radio interviews of influenza experts. Tommy Thompson, former Secretary of the U.S. Department of Health and Human Services, made an interesting comment at a news conference he gave just before departing his office in early December 2004. He said that one of the things he was very concerned about was a worldwide influenza pandemic that could result in the deaths of 30 to 70 million people. Officially, however, the government is standing by their rosy scenarios.

In my view, the gross underestimate of the impact of the next pandemic on the United States by the Department of Health and Human Services suggests a number of unsavory possibilities. Since they have access to the best-educated and brightest epidemiologists and medical scientists, the reason for their less than robust prediction is not for lack of information or analytic ability. It is likely that the forces and motives operating within the U.S. government that lead to this treatment of the truth are shared by other national governments as well.

What the Government Is Doing to Stop It

Vaccines

Vaccination is the most effective method of protecting against this infection. Overall, vaccination is considered 70 percent effective in prevention of influenza. The most commonly employed method of flu vaccine manufacture entails growing live virus in fertilized chicken eggs and then separating the viral particles from the egg. The particles are inactivated by heat, blended, and then mixed with sterile water to produce a specific concentration of killed viral particle proteins. Purified killed influenza vaccine is proven to be safe and effective for producing protection against flu infection.

The composition of the annual flu vaccine changes every year to include the strains that are circulating in the human population. The World Health Organization makes recommendations twice a year, and the ultimate composition of the vaccine is decided by the national health authority in each country. For instance, in the U.S., the decision rests with an advisory committee of the Food and Drug Administration. Typically, for seasonal

---

How Does a Vaccine Protect You?

When you receive a vaccine, your body's immune system recognizes these viral proteins as foreign invaders and mounts a vigorous campaign to destroy them by making antibodies to fight them and others that search out and destroy the virus directly.

These cells remain on alert in your body, on guard for any sign that influenza has invaded. If they detect the strain of influenza that they recognize, they are called into action: They multiply rapidly and quickly mount a usually successful defense.

One common misconception about flu vaccination is that it prevents infection with flu entirely. This is not so. You can be infected with the flu even if you've been successfully vaccinated against that strain of flu; however, if you've been vaccinated, the resulting infection is much milder and shorter in duration, and resembles a cold more than the flu. Some vaccinated patients have no symptoms at all when they contract the flu.

---

flu, the United States orders 90 million doses, enough to immunize all who fit the CDC's recommended list for flu vaccination. This includes the very young, the elderly, the infirm, healthcare workers, public safety officers and all adults age fifty and older. There is very little vaccine earmarked for healthy teens or younger adults.

Limited Vaccine Supply

Today, world influenza vaccine capacity is just 300 million doses—only enough to protect 5 percent of the world's population. Obviously, with the world's population now exceeding 6.6 billion, when the next pandemic occurs, there won't be enough vaccine to go around. In an article in the July/August 2005 issue of *Foreign Affairs*, Michael Osterholm notes: "Even if the system functions to the best of its ability, influenza vaccine is produced commercially in just nine countries: Australia, Canada, France, Germany, Italy, Japan, the Netherlands, the United Kingdom and the United States. These countries contain only 12 percent of the world's population. In the event of an influenza pandemic, they would probably nationalize their domestic production facilities, as occurred in 1976, when the United States, anticipating a pandemic of swine influenza (H1N1), refused to share its vaccine."

Stretching the Supply

Recent studies show that young, healthy adults can become immune with a reduced (half) dose of killed flu protein if it is given combined with an *adjuvant*, a substance that stimulates the immune response to a protein. By mixing the vaccine supply with an adjuvant, we could roughly double the current supply, but even that would not be nearly enough to protect the world's population. Some experts have advocated that the world's flu vaccine be shared more equitably between the developed (G8) countries that are now slated to get 90 percent of the vaccine output and the rest of the world. It does not appear that there will be a marked increase in vaccine manufacturing capacity or sharing of the limited vaccine supply.

In March 2005, Sanofi Pasteur, the French vaccine manufacturer, released the first vaccine made for humans directed against the avian influenza A H5N1 virus for testing and evaluation by virology laboratories. This virus was based on a version of the virus that was circulating in 2004. Tests showed it was effective, but in a much higher than usual dose, meaning that fewer immunizations could be given from the same amount of vaccine. Additional testing of adjuvants to extend the vaccine supply is also underway. While vaccine production using fertilized eggs takes six to eight months under the best of circumstances, it has been more difficult than usual with the H5N1 strain because it is so lethal that it kills the chicken embryo before there is enough time raise a good yield of viable particles. New methods of producing vaccines are needed and are being discussed and, in some cases, developed.

The Sanofi Pasteur H5N1 avian flu vaccine is unlikely to be of much use against the virus that eventually evolves as a human threat. Because the flu virus is always changing, both spontaneously and by swapping genetic material with other viruses when both infect the same organism, it constitutes an unpredictably moving target for the vaccine makers. Since it is impossible to predict what the pandemic flu will look like before it emerges, the planned vaccine for next season is highly unlikely to provide any protection against the pandemic avian influenza strain.

While vaccination is our best hope of avoiding catastrophe, it's fairly certain that none will be available when the first wave of the pandemic spreads across the globe. This means that in all likelihood, the first wave will be characterized with a high rate of infection and many deaths. The time between the first and second wave is crucial because there needs to be enough time for the flu manufacturers to brew enough vaccine to protect as many of the remaining susceptible population as possible. Patients who contract the flu during the first wave and live, will in all likelihood be immune from the pandemic strain, so they won't need to be vaccinated. This includes those who become infected with pandemic flu, become ill, and are successfully treated with the antiviral drugs Tamiflu or Relenza.

Antiviral Drugs—Scarce Yet Effective . . . for Now

The World Health Organization has recommended that every country establish a stockpile of enough drugs to treat 20 percent of its citizens in preparation for a possible avian influenza pandemic. Most of the developed nations have begun to do so, the U.S. more slowly than most. In late May 2005, Roche's medical director for Tamiflu testified to a House of Representatives subcommittee that the United States' "stockpile purchases to date are sufficient to treat less than 1 percent of the U.S. population. We have also received a non-binding letter of intent for HHS to purchase additional treatments to cover under 2 percent of the population. In contrast, countries such as the United Kingdom, France, Finland, Norway, Switzerland and New Zealand are ordering enough Tamiflu to cover between 20 to 40 percent of their populations. . . . Any government that does not stockpile sufficient quantities of Tamiflu in advance cannot be assured of an adequate supply at the outbreak of a pandemic."[6]

Tamiflu

The antiviral drug tablet, Tamiflu® (oseltamivir) manufactured by Roche Pharmaceuticals, is effective against avian influenza H5N1. The wholesale cost of Tamiflu is about $25 for a five-day treatment course (ten tablets), a price that places it out of reach for the less developed nations to establish a Tamiflu stockpile. Manufacturing capacity for Tamiflu is also limited and takes place almost entirely in Europe. Most of the G8 countries have already placed their orders with Roche and governmental demand has been so great that this product was unavailable for a while in the spring of 2005; as of June 2005, Tamiflu began to trickle back into the retail chain but supplies remain tight.

Tamiflu works best if it is taken within the first forty-eight hours of the onset of symptoms. It might be useful even if started later but this is not established. In the event of a pandemic, I plan to administer Tamiflu to very sick patients no matter how long they have had symptoms as long as there is hope they can survive.

It is also possible to prevent the flu by taking Tamiflu tablets at or immediately after exposure to the flu. While this strategy works, it requires the continuous use of the one tablet daily until the pandemic is past. Given the critical shortage of Tamiflu that we would likely face during a pandemic, using the drug in this way is unwise. The strategy I plan to follow is to wait until flu symptoms are present before beginning Tamiflu treatment. The recommended dose is one tablet twice daily for five days. However, a worrisome U.S. National Institute of Health study published in the July 2005 issue of the *Journal of Infectious Disease*[7] reported that mice experimentally infected with the H5N1 avian flu strain required ten days of Tamiflu treatment to prevent relapse and death instead of the currently recommended five-day course. If this proves true for the pandemic virus, it means patients would need treatment for ten days to survive. This is a big problem since the current stock of this drug would go only half as far as thought initially.

The good news concerning antiviral supply is that studies of influenza antibody levels in people before and after influenza epidemics reveal that the percentage of patients with blood evidence of having had the flu is twice as high as the reported clinical attack rate for the epidemic. In other words, for every person who gets sick with the flu there is another person who contracts the virus but has no or very few symptoms of the illness. This means, in the event of a pandemic, even if you don't take Tamiflu in the preventive regimen you still have a 50 percent chance of not getting sick. By reserving the drug for those who become ill with flu, you will be able to effectively treat a much larger number of patients than if the drug is used in its preventive mode.

The bad news is, as reported in May 2005, some strains of H5N1 avian influenza that have crossed over from birds to humans in Southeast Asia that are developing resistance to Tamiflu. A report published in *Nature* magazine states that a Vietnamese girl had a case of the avian flu that was resistant to Tamiflu.[8]

While this is a disturbing observation, it doesn't mean that if the pandemic flu arrives in the United States it will be totally resistant to Tamiflu treatment. It's likely, however, that some strains of the virus will carry this resistance factor; meaning that some patients infected by those strains will not respond to Tamiflu as well as expected.

Relenza

There's a second antiviral drug, Relenza° (zanamivir) that has been shown to be effective against some strains of the H5N1 avian flu. Relenza has not been as much of a commercial success as Tamiflu because it is a powder that is inhaled through a mouth-piece, and therefore not as convenient. Avian flu has been found to be resistant to the other older anti-influenza drugs like aman-tadine. So, other than a specific vaccine that has not yet been pro-duced, and the antiviral drugs Tamiflu and Relenza, there really isn't much else that can be done medically to prepare for this event. Our limited options are exactly why you need to learn other ways to protect you and your family with a pre-pandemic plan.

Practical Pre-Pandemic Preparations for Individuals

In the event of a major pandemic with a case fatality rate that exceeds 5 percent, it's likely there will be a temporary breakdown in food delivery, the electric and water utility services, and possibly even public order in urban areas worldwide. This prediction is based on several factors. First is the marked expansion in the human population since the last major pandemic. In 1918, our population was 1.6 billion; today it's 6.6 billion. In 1918, only 17 percent of the world's inhabitants lived in urban environments, and there were only fifteen cities with more than one million inhabitants. Today, there are over 400 cities with a population of more than one million people.[9] The difficulty is not in predicting whether these population factors will worsen or lessen the severity of the pandemic. There is no question that it will worsen it, but by how much, we don't know.

Cities are dependent on outside sources for critical supplies including food, power and water. The provision of these essential goods and services requires the highly coordinated efforts of a large number of people. During a major pandemic, these activities are likely to be interrupted by widespread illness and death. The interdependent nature of modern society increases the risk that a systematic failure could occur due to a domino effect precipitated by the failures of one or two key institutions or resources. In other words, a failure of one critical system leads to the failure of another and so on until the entire system collapses.

Taken together, these factors are likely to produce a temporary disruption in the basic supplies and services we all now take for granted. The resulting chaos would likely be accompanied by a period of temporary anarchy, especially within large urban centers.

My estimate is that when H5N1 avian flu crosses over there is a one out of three chance of a major pandemic and a two out of three chance of a minor one. The most likely time for this to happen now is between December 2005 and March 2006.[10] If we have a major event, it would be prudent to plan to be self-reliant for about three months. The question is, how?

Get Your Will in Order

Let's face it; you might not make it through a major pandemic. It is likely that one in forty won't. So, get your will in order. Make sure you have a plan for those surviving that will see them through.

Make Sure You Have Life Insurance

If you need to, buy more life insurance now since it takes time to get a policy. If nothing happens, you can always cancel it later.

You may wish to consider buying a life insurance policy for your spouse and children. It would be prudent to select only the bluest of blue chip insurers, as the economic impact of a major pandemic will not be predictable.

Get a Flu Shot and a Pneumovax Vaccination

Even though the vaccine for the 2005-6 flu season does not include protection against the avian flu, I recommend you get one. The reason for this is that many experts predict that the most likely time for the pandemic to begin is during the regular flu season. If you get the flu shot, it will protect you against the seasonal flu and prevent you from developing it during the same time that pandemic flu is circulating in your community. Also, you do not want to come down with flu twice in the same year. Since pandemic flu is so different antigenically than seasonal flu, this could happen; and if it does, your chances of surviving the second infection are worse, especially if you're still weakened by the first one. You can protect yourself from pneumococcal pneumonia, a potential flu complication, by getting a Pneumovax vaccination. This will be important in the event that we experience a major flu pandemic. I recommend these immunizations for adults and children.

Prepare a Stockpile of Food and Other Necessities

In the event of a major pandemic, food supplies are likely to become limited. Storing a supply of canned meat and fish, dried beans and rice is a prudent consideration. Consider basics like salt, sugar, cooking oil, and multiple vitamins as well. If food shipments are interrupted to the cities, it won't be very long before food is gone from the grocery shelves. If you have any doubt about this, think about what happens when there is a threat of a hurricane or snowstorm. (See the list of bare essentials on the following page. Some of these items are listed in detail in the Flu Survival Kit on page 34.)

Medical Supplies

❑ Thermometer (more than one)

❑ Blood pressure monitor

❑ Notebook

❑ Measuring cup

❑ Medicine dropper

❑ BandAids

❑ Gauze pads

❑ Tissues

❑ Toilet paper

Over-the-Counter Medicines

❑ Ibuprofen

❑ Acetaminophen

❑ Benadryl

❑ Tums Ex

❑ Cough syrup or suppressant

❑ Vitamins

❑ Antibiotic ointment

Prescription Medicines

❑ Refills of prescriptions for family members

❑ Tamiflu (or Relenza)

❏ Promethazine
❏ Hydrocodone with acetaminophen
❏ Diazepam

Cleaning Agents

❏ Bleach
❏ Disinfectant
❏ Instant hand sanitizer

Food/Pantry Items

❏ Sugar
❏ Table salt
❏ Baking soda
❏ Water
❏ Juice
❏ Pedialyte or Gatorade
❏ Caffeinated tea, dry loose
❏ Ice
❏ White toast
❏ White rice
❏ Cream of wheat
❏ Soda crackers
❏ Potatoes

☐ Milk
☐ Butter
☐ Rice
☐ Dry beans
☐ Canned fruits and vegetables
☐ Canned meats and fish
☐ Solar-powered batteries
☐ Flashlights
☐ Shortwave Radio

Consider Alternative Power Sources

The United States power grid is fragile, especially on the east and west coasts. Despite the brown and blackouts of 2003, not much has been done to reduce the power grid's vulnerability, the energy bill of July 2005 notwithstanding. Since it's literally interconnected, what happens in one part impacts another. While the grid has some built-in automatic circuit breakers designed to isolate a power overload condition before it spreads and causes a widespread blackout, for the most part, the system is operator dependent.

Much of the power production in the United States is coal-fired, and these units depend upon regular delivery of coal by rail. Power industry guidelines call for the plants to keep at least a twenty-five-day coal stockpile to ensure uninterrupted power production in the event of a supply disruption. If a critical number of system engineers (employed by the plant, the railroad, or the coalmine) become ill, die, or are otherwise absent as a result of the pandemic, the plants would shut down. Nuclear plants could also be shut down if the number of personnel fell below a predefined threshold for safe operation.

Since plant and grid repair and restart crews would also be affected in a similar manner to the engineers, the time to bring the shutdown system back up would also be more prolonged than under normal conditions. If enough plants were affected, the chances of brownouts or blackouts affecting large regions could be prolonged.

Interruptions in electric power service could last a month or two or more. One way to cope with this potential problem is to buy a small supply of essential battery operated devices like lighting, flashlights and a radio. Nickel Metal Hydride (NiMH) rechargeable batteries are now available that are a much-improved rechargeable battery compared with what was available in the past. In addition, you can find a wide selection of solar-powered battery chargers. These chargers can be coupled with a photovoltaic (solar power) module that will reliably and quickly (if big enough) charge your NiMH batteries over and over again. Good NiMH batteries, various chargers, and a selection of small PV modules suitable for this purpose can be purchased from Real Goods at *www.realgoods.com*.

Prepare a Source of Drinkable Water

In the event of a pandemic, you could expect that the operational staff at public water systems would experience illness at the average rate of the community as a whole. So, absenteeism could affect service reliability, as would loss of electric power, because these utilities use electric pumps to pressurize their systems. If water service is interrupted for a time, remember to wait a while before drinking the water once service is restored because it may be contaminated with bacteria initially. Before that, you can boil it or add 1/8 teaspoon of household bleach to each gallon of water to purify it.

It would be wise to store some potable (drinkable) water to use in case of emergency. Ideally you should try to have a gallon of water a day per person. You can store tap water in fifty-five-gallon drums. Make sure the drum you purchase is new; if not, make sure that it is safe to use for storing drinking water and that it didn't at one time hold toxic chemicals. You might also consider how you could divert rainwater from your downspouts for storage and drinking. Water collected from the roof will need to be purified before drinking because it could be contaminated. I found several helpful water purification suggestions on the US Federal Emergency Management Administration's web site.[11]

Communicate with the Outside World

Local TV and radio broadcasts would probably cease if there was a regional power failure in your area as would cable TV. Satellite TV may remain active but you would need an alternative source of power to operate your system since your power would be out. Landline telephone systems have an excellent record of remaining operational even during power failures.

However, in the event of a widespread prolonged blackout, they will not be able to function for very long. Cell phone towers have a small backup power capability but this won't last long. So if the grid fails, all phone service will as well.

A good quality battery operated radio capable of receiving AM, FM, and Short Wave stations would be a smart way to keep up with local and world events in the event that the usual methods were impaired. Even if there are no operative local or regional news broadcasts, someone somewhere will be on the air reporting information of interest to flu survivors. It will be comforting having access to this information should a major pandemic come to pass.

Find a Rural Refuge

During the Spanish Flu pandemic, those who fled from centers of population were safer than those who stayed, but even small communities were hit hard so location offers no guarantee of safety. By 1919 the flu had hit about every community, so living in a rural area is not going to be enough. Reverse quarantines—keeping outsiders from entering and bringing the flu with them—did work occasionally in 1918. Some small communities might try this approach in modern times, but for any hope of success, reverse quarantines will need to be very strict and started at the outset of a pandemic or they will not work.

One lesson from major epidemics is that these events almost always lead to civil disorder. For this reason alone it would be wise to ride out the storm away from cities or other major population centers. It's probable that food and water will be easier to obtain in the country and people will be less hostile compared with what can be imagined in the major metropolitan areas.

If you plan to leave the city for the country, you should do so early in the pandemic. President Bush said in an October 4, 2005 news conference that he was considering imposing reverse quarantines in the event of a pandemic. If you plan to remain where you live now during the pandemic, then prepare your home. If not, then prepare the place you plan to stay. You need to be ready to move fast should the flu hit the United States. My advice is to, at minimum, secure the items listed in the Flu Survival Kit on page 34; enough for each family member. These items should be kept in a specific location where you can quickly get your hands on them.

Hospital and Healthcare Services

In the event of a major pandemic, healthcare services, especially hospital services, will be rapidly overwhelmed; in fact, it's likely that the healthcare system will be the first societal institution to collapse under the strain, with recovery not expected until after the return of other essential utilities and services. The first victims of the flu will get excellent treatment, including hospitalization and even ventilators if required. Before long, though, all the available resources will be exhausted.

In order to reduce healthcare costs, hospitals have significantly reduced the number of available patient beds and nursing staff.

It's a common occurrence today for hospitals to be "on bypass" when it comes to accepting critically ill patients in their emergency rooms via ambulance. This happens when every ICU and CCU bed is already occupied. During a routine flu season, it's not uncommon to find that most every critical care bed and available ventilator in many U.S. cities are fully occupied for weeks each year. You can imagine that if the number of critically ill patients presenting to hospital emergency departments with pulmonary failure from influenza suddenly increased exponentially over those with the seasonal flu, the chances of getting an ICU bed or ventilator would be nil. Once the pandemic settles in, the hospitals will be overloaded to capacity, including waiting rooms and hallways. The medical staff will be sick themselves; some will be dead. The hospital will quickly run out of supplies and there will be a shortage of everything from drugs and bandages to IV fluids and body bags. So, in my opinion, it would be unwise to remain in the city so you can take advantage of the healthcare system in case you become ill.

Stocking Your Survival Kit

Even under "normal" circumstances, it's a good idea to have a supply of over-the-counter products and select prescription drugs on hand for home treatment of influenza. Under extraordinarily trying conditions, it is essential to life.

For instance, simple household items that can make a big difference to health include ibuprofen, acetaminophen, table sugar and table salt. See the list of home essentials on page 25; the time to secure these items is before you need them—hopefully you will not. If you find the list too daunting, break it down into small shopping trips or buy some of the items online.

It will also be helpful to have on hand, and know how to use a thermometer, an automatic blood pressure and pulse monitor. In the following discussion I will provide you with advice on how these simple items can be used very effectively for the home care of flu sufferers. In order to obtain the prescription drugs needed for the home care of the flu, please call your doctor who is best able to advise you. I have included the over-the-counter and prescription items that I think will be most useful but your doctor may have other equally good or better suggestions especially since he or she knows your specific medical condition much better than anyone else.

Flu Survival Kit

The following over-the-counter products are useful for home treatment of one person with severe influenza:

- ❏ Table salt: 1 lb
- ❏ Table sugar: 10 lbs
- ❏ Baking soda: 6 oz
- ❏ Household bleach 1 gal[12]
- ❏ Tums Ex: 500 tablets
- ❏ Acetaminophen 500mg #100 tablets
- ❏ Ibuprofen 200mg # 100 tablets
- ❏ Caffeinated tea, dry loose: 1 lb
- ❏ Electronic thermometer: #2[13]
- ❏ Automatic blood pressure monitor[14]
- ❏ Notebook to record vital signs and fluid intake and output
- ❏ Kitchen measuring cup with 500 cc (two cup) capacity
- ❏ Diphenhydramine (Benadryl) 25mg capsules # 60: 1 tablet every 4 hours as needed for nasal congestion, allergy or itching.

The following prescriptions products are useful for home treatment of one person with severe influenza:

- ❏ Tamiflu 75mg # 20: take two tablets daily for 5 (or 10) days for flu[15]
- ❏ Promethazine (Phenergan) 25mg tablets # 60: take 1/2 to 1 tablet every 4 hrs as needed for nausea
- ❏ Hydrocodone with acetaminophen (Lortab-5) # 60 (5mg/325mg): 1/2 to 1 tablet every 4 hrs as needed for cough or pain
- ❏ Diazepam (Valium) 5mg # 60: 1/2 to 1 tablet twice daily as needed for anxiety, muscle aches or insomnia

Simple Medical Skills Required

Caregivers need to learn how to obtain vital signs like pulse, blood pressure, temperature and respiratory rate. It will also be very useful to be able to use an automated blood pressure monitor to measure blood pressure. These devices come with pretty good instructions that clearly explain how to use them. "Practice makes perfect" applies to learning and perfecting these skills. If you need help learning how to do these, ask your doctor or his or her nurse for help. They will be happy to help you develop these simple skills. All you need to do is ask.

Symptoms of Influenza

The influenza virus usually enters the body through the respiratory tract but can also gain access through the intestinal tract. The most common symptoms are fever, sore throat, cough, runny nose and general aches and pains; it may also cause headache, nausea, abdominal cramps and diarrhea.

If people are experiencing some of these symptoms, it doesn't necessarily mean they are infected with the avian flu virus: Their symptoms could be due to another infectious agent or even the influenza virus but not the avian strain, since it's possible that both endemic (routine seasonal flu varieties) and pandemic strains could both be circulating in the community at the same time. In fact, this scenario is entirely possible.

A Cold or the Flu?

There are several ways to tell the difference between the flu and less severe illnesses. First of all, unless the flu is circulating in the community, then your illness is probably not flu, because it tends to occur in epidemics that are easy to spot epidemiologically. If the world is in the midst of a major pandemic, you will have no problem knowing about it. Just tune into CNN, or another national news outlet, as it is likely to be pandemic coverage 24/7. Another clue to whether or not someone has flu is that flu is much worse than a simple cold virus or most other causes of respiratory or gastrointestinal (GI) infections. The fever and body aches are really quite remarkable and often associated with strong shivering.

When flu affects the GI tract it presents with nausea, vomiting and diarrhea. Patients with flu are really sick and often are so weak they have a hard time getting up out of bed without help. So, one way to tell the difference between the flu and other infections is that the flu is really severe and tends to affect the respiratory track most often, but can also cause severe gastroenteritis (nausea, vomiting, and diarrhea).

Patient Prognosis During Pandemic Influenza

One difference between a major pandemic flu and the annual flu is how hard it hits patients and how rapidly it kills. Patients affected by pandemic flu can be broadly categorized into three prognostic types. The first type has a poor prognosis no matter what is done for them. The second type might survive if there was full access to high-technology medical care and resources. The third type is highly likely to recover from the flu as long as they are provided with consistent low-technology supportive measures that can be administered in home settings.

Type 1 patients have the poorest prognosis and almost all will die within two or three days after development of their first symptoms. The cause of death in these patients during the 1918 flu was massive respiratory failure from viral pneumonia that overwhelmed their lungs. There was no effective treatment for this in 1918, and there is none today despite all the advances in medicine that have occurred over the last nearly ninety years. Signs and symptoms of type 1 patients include rapid onset of severe shortness of breath, cyanosis (bluish discoloration of the skin of the hands, feet, and around the mouth and spreading centrally), or bleeding from the lungs, stomach and rectum.

Type 2 patients are similar to type 1 patients except they are ill for a longer period of time. Some—but not many—of these patients would survive if they had access to an ICU, ventilators and expert medical care, resources that will not be widely available if we have a major pandemic. Even if they had access to these services, many of these patients would die, usually within a week to ten days after becoming ill.

Type 3 patients make up the majority of those that become ill with influenza. Fortunately, these patients have a good prognosis if they receive timely and diligent supportive care that can be provided well in a non-medical setting such as the home. Most of these flu victims will be severely ill and so weakened by the infection that they will not be able to get out of bed. Many type 3 patients will be completely dependent on others for care. Without simple care, some of these patients will die from preventable causes like dehydration but with simple care, most of these patients will recover. No matter how good the care provided, some type 3 patients will die. This is not your fault. This happens usually because they develop a serious secondary condition that actually becomes the cause of death. Examples of these secondary conditions include bacterial pneumonia, stroke and heart attack. There is nothing you can do but keep doing your best and let nature take its course.

In my opinion, as a general rule, provide everyone with the same level of supportive care. This is a rational course because it is not always possible to predict who will survive and who will not, especially early in the course of the flu.

Using Scarce Resources Wisely

Patients *in extremis*, which means they are near death at the time they are encountered, should not be disturbed unless there is something that you can do to make them more comfortable. Fortunately, patients *in extremis* are usually already unconscious and beyond suffering.

If medical supplies are in short supply, especially the antiviral drug Tamiflu, the decision on how to ration these resources is best made by health professionals if they are available. If not, my

READER/CUSTOMER CARE SURVEY

HEFM

We care about your opinions! Please take a moment to fill out our online Reader Survey at
http://survey.hcibooks.com. As a **"THANK YOU"** you will receive a **VALUABLE INSTANT COUPON** towards future
book purchases as well as a **SPECIAL GIFT** available only online! Or, you may mail this card back to us
and we will send you a copy of our exciting catalog with your valuable coupon inside.

First Name _____ M.I. _____ Last Name _____

Address _____ Email _____

State _____ Zip _____ City _____

1. Gender	**4. Annual**	**6. Marital Status**
❏ Female ❏ Male	**Household Income**	❏ Single
	❏ under $25,000	❏ Married
2. Age	❏ $25,000 - $34,999	❏ Divorced
❏ 8 or younger	❏ $35,000 - $49,999	❏ Widowed
❏ 9-12 ❏ 13-16	❏ $50,000 - $74,999	
❏ 17-20 ❏ 21-30	❏ over $75,000	**Comments**
❏ 31+		
	5. What are the	
3. Did you receive	**ages of the children**	
this book as a gift?	**living in your house?**	
❏ Yes ❏ No	❏ 0 - 14 ❏ 15+	

BUSINESS REPLY MAIL

FIRST-CLASS MAIL PERMIT NO 45 DEERFIELD BEACH, FL

POSTAGE WILL BE PAID BY ADDRESSEE

Health Communications, Inc.

3201 SW 15th Street

Deerfield Beach FL 33442-9875

suggestion is to concentrate your efforts and precious supplies on those with the best chance of survival, i.e., type 3 patients. In a severe pandemic it is unwise to use limited medical resources on critically ill type 1 or 2 patients, as they are unlikely to survive. So my advice is to focus your greatest efforts on type 3 patients where the prognosis is good for a complete recovery.

Home Flu Treatment Advice for the Layperson

Caring for severely ill flu patients is something that everyone is capable of doing. No advanced medical skills are required. The skills needed are the same one parents use to care for their young children or adult children use to care for their elderly parents. The basic goals are to keep the patient clean, dry, warm and well hydrated. The patient needs a comfortable place to lie down and they need to be told that they are going to be okay, and reassured that you will be there for them. *The most important medical treatment is to make sure they have plenty of fluids. Dehydration must be prevented, as this can be fatal in a patient who would otherwise survive.* Remember: Keeping the patient hydrated is the best treatment for the flu and the one most likely to save lives.

What to Do for Fever, Body Aches, Chills, Sore Throat and Headache

Ibuprofen and/or acetaminophen is effective treatment for these symptoms; both can lower fever and help the patient feel better. Use these products for the flu according to my instructions, not the bottle label; in other words, don't under-dose the patient. Many people take doses that are ineffective for fear of taking too much. Acetaminophen can be used at the same time, and in full doses, as ibuprofen because they are in different drug classes and therefore have different drug side effects. Combination treatment with both has an additive effect of benefit without increasing risk. The dose of ibuprofen I recommend you use is 2 to 4 tablets (400mg to 800mg) every four hours.[16] For acetaminophen, the dose is two 500mg tablets 4 times daily. **Do not exceed these doses for either drug.** This is the maximum for both. There is a risk of causing Reyes Syndrome if children and teens with fever are given aspirin or aspirin like drugs including ibuprofen. Reyes is a rare occurrence (1:1,000,000 annually) but can be fatal. Reyes is associated with increased pressure in the brain and liver damage. When confronted with a child or teen with an unremitting high fever (more than 104 degrees F) that is not responding to acetaminophen/hydration/and tepid-water sponge baths, one has to consider the risk of brain damage from fever versus risk from Reyes. This is a tough call. I would probably use the aspirin in this case, understanding various risks.

A very high fever (more than 104 degrees F) can cause seizures and brain damage and must be avoided. Tepid-water sponge baths work well to bring down a high fever. Do not use alcohol sponge baths instead of water. Alcohol can be absorbed through the skin, especially in children, resulting in toxic effects. Ibuprofen and acetaminophen are very good at lowering temperature. Studies show that the body's natural defenses are better able to fight infection with some fever (say up to 101 degrees F), so don't try to completely suppress the temperature to normal (98.6 degrees F).

Gargling with hot salt water is a good treatment for sore throat. Hot caffeinated tea is also very helpful for headache, sore throat and cough (caffeine has long been recognized for its pharmacologic effect as an excellent herbal therapy). Hot or cold tea is also a mild stimulant that improves the sense of the patient's well-being. Sore throats also respond well to ibuprofen or acetaminophen.

The Patient's Diet

The flu takes the appetite away, so the patient probably won't be hungry. Don't worry, eating is not really important because the patient will be breaking down their own muscle and fat for energy. If the patient is hungry and asks for food, this is great sign of improvement. By all means feed the patient at that point, but your food selection needs to be appropriate. See specific directions on how to feed patients recovering from severe flu on page 50.

Fluids

What will be much appreciated by a sick patient, especially if they are dehydrated, is a simple Oral Rehydration Solution (ORS) made from water, sugar and salt.

The ORS Formula

ORS is simply homemade IV fluids for oral use. You can use it for flu patients and those with diarrhea and even cholera. It is better than plain water for dehydrated patients, because the body needs the salt, and the sugar helps the water enter and remain in the body. It's the same principle as a sports drink like Gatorade. Water is much better than nothing, but the ORS formula is better than water. The formula is:

4 cups of clean water
3 tablespoons of sugar or honey
¼ tsp table salt[17, 18]

Identifying Dehydration

Preventing dehydration in flu victims will save more lives than all the other treatments combined. When patients have a fever or diarrhea, they lose much more water from the body than people realize. Symptoms of dehydration include weakness, headache and fainting and tell-tale signs include dryness of the mouth, decreased saliva, lack of or very decreased urine that is dark and highly concentrated, sunken eyes, loss of skin turgor (the elasticity of the skin), low blood pressure especially upon sitting up or rising from the sitting to the standing position and tachycardia (fast pulse) when laying or sitting up.

Fever is an especially easy way to become dehydrated without anyone noticing because fluid can escape through the skin and quickly evaporate. This is called *insensible loss,* and great quantities of fluid can escape a patient quickly this way. The smaller the patient's body size and the higher the temperature, the faster this can happen. Water in the form of vapor is also lost through breathing, so when the patient is short of breath and breathing rapidly, this is another source of hidden fluid loss.

Pushing Fluids

If you suspect that dehydration is developing, administer fluids by mouth. If the patient is too ill to drink, someone should sit with the patient and give him fluids drop by drop if needed, working up to using a teaspoon if possible. Don't stop until the patient keeps down at least a quart of fluids. This could take several hours so be patient. It will have a dramatic effect on a sick patient and will be very rewarding to you because your actions may well save a life. After the first quart, the patient should begin to urinate again. This is a good prognostic sign: when this happens you can assume you have restored their fluid level back to a safer level. "Safer" should not be confused with safe. Don't stop there. With sick patients like these, you really need to "push the fluids," so don't let your guard down.

You can serve fluids cool or hot, depending on the climate, patient symptoms and fever status. A patient with a high fever should probably not be given hot fluids because it will raise the temperature further. A patient hot with fever might prefer a cool or even cold beverage. A patient with a sore throat will get relief from a hot beverage. If it is cold outside, especially if the patient is cold, use hot fluids. You can give the ORS plain or flavor it with just about anything like citrus, mint or herbs.

If juice is available, you can substitute 1 cup of it for 1 cup of the water and cut the sweetener in half. Boil the solution to purify it if needed or you can purify water for drinking by adding 1/8 teaspoon of household bleach to 1 gallon of water. Administering fluids to the sick in your charge will be one of the main activities day in and day out until the crisis passes. Try to get 2 to 3 quarts of fluids down the patient every day at a minimum. Don't give up or slack off. Make this your most important task.

Preventing Germs from Spreading in Your Household

It is unlikely that we will be able to limit exposure to the virus if there are a lot of sick people around us. The flu is so easily passed from one person to the next that it is difficult to control even in hospitals. The WHO has issued guidelines for reducing exposure among healthcare workers taking care of rare cases of H5N1 flu under "non-pandemic" conditions in the hospital setting. It is not likely that these techniques will be able to be followed for very long after the pandemic gets going, especially in the case of a major pandemic. The WHO recommendations were published in the September 28, 2005 issue of the *New England Journal of Medicine*.[19] Under these pre-pandemic conditions the WHO recommends such things as negative pressure rooms, long-sleeved full-length gowns, gloves, and NIOSH N-95 masks, face shields or eye goggles.

Obviously these recommendations are not appropriate for home care. In truth, pandemic influenza is so infectious that people who are taking care of sick folks in our homes are simply not going to be able to prevent being exposed to the virus. As we provide needed care to our family, friends and even sick strangers we will be constantly exposed to infectious viral particles. This will happen when we change soiled patient clothes and bedclothes and clean up food and drink and tissues. Simply breathing the air in the vicinity of the sick person will result in significant exposure, which is why setting up one "sick room" in the house can be effective in reducing exposure to all family members. Using a cloth facemask is not effective in preventing exposure; however when worn it's useful for preventing you from spreading disease to someone else. Masks were thought to be an effective means of preventing spread of bacterial pneumonia as secondary infections in patients with lungs already weakened by flu during the 1918 pandemic but this opinion was never proven scientifically.

It will be very important to keep the sick and their bed and bed clothing clean and dry. Likewise the sick rooms and bathrooms need to be maintained in good condition. Any soiled garments and bed-clothes, as well as contaminated bedding, will need to be washed and dried, a task likely to be made quite challenging by the possible lack of electrical and water service. It will be important to wash any contaminated items in hot water using soap and chlorine bleach if possible. Disinfectant household hard surfaces by wiping them clean using soap and water and then spraying them with 1:10 bleach to water solution; wipe them down a second time. This disinfecting regime will effectively remove all trace harmful germs and particles.

While it will be difficult—if not impossible—to shield caregivers from exposure given their close contact with patients, if this pandemic behaves as expected, roughly half of us will *not* develop symptoms of flu; if we do, we will have mild cases. Those of us who do develop infection and recover will be immune from the pandemic strain in the future.

Keep a Record on Every Patient

It will be very useful for you to write down certain information about the patient or patients you are taking care of at home. Devote a section of the notebook to each patient. Keep the record in chronological order day by day, being as accurate as you can. Don't worry about keeping a perfect record; just keep one as best you can using the following as a sample guide.

Each morning, take the patient's vital signs. Include their temperature, pulse rate, breathing rate and blood pressure. Repeat the vital signs routinely four times daily (for instance at 8:00, 12:00, 4:00, and 6:00). You should measure these vital signs more often in very sick patients. Keeping records on the patient's fluid intake and output is very important. Intake is fairly easy since you are giving them the fluids but output can be difficult to accurately record. Have the patients save all their urine by urinating in a bucket, pot, or basin instead of the toilet. Measure the urine output using the kitchen measuring cup. The amount taken in is always more than the amount output passed out because of the insensible losses described above (loss through the skin and in the breath). If the patient is incontinent of urine, just indicate in the record that the patient was incontinent of a small, medium or large amount of urine. For our purposes, large is good, small is bad.

Example Home Patient Medical Record

Patient Name: Mary Smith

Date of Birth: 3-31-1951

Date symptoms first began: January 15, 2006

1-17-05 3:00 PM Initial Note

Subjective (S)[20]: Mary became weak and faint today after suffering from muscle aches and pains for the last couple of days. She has trouble standing up without dizziness. She is nauseated and also complains of headache and sore throat. She is urinating but not as much as usual. She has been trying to drink more but has been busy taking care of the sick. She has not been getting much sleep for the last 2 weeks.

Objective (O): Vital Signs: Temp: 102 F[21], Pulse: 110/min and regular[22], Resp Rate: 22/min[23], BP 100/60[24] The skin is pale and mildly moist. Mary looks very tired but is awake and alert. Her mouth is moist.

Assessment (A): Flu with mild dehydration and fatigue

Plan (P): Push fluids (ORS), ibuprofen 800 mg every 4 hours as needed for temp > 101 or pain. Bed rest. Keep track of fluid intake and urine output. Take VS and check hydration, fluid input/output, and 4 times daily. (Begin Tamifu if you have it.) (Use anti-nausea meds if available.)

1-17-05 6:30 PM
Subjective—(what the patient tells you) Mary's sleeping on and off. She feels less faint but still dizzy. She is peeing.
Objective—what you record and observe) Temp 100 F, Pulse 90/min, BP 100/60
Fluid In: 1500 ml[25] ORS, Urine Out: 250 ml
A-your assessment of condition) Flu, improved symptoms, patient still dehydrated but hydration underway
P-your plan to make the patient better) Push more fluids.

Diet Recommendations

The Clear Liquid Diet

A clear liquid diet is used to treat certain intestinal diseases, especially infectious diarrhea. Patients suffering from diarrheal illnesses often experience abdominal cramping and frequent, loose stools if they eat solid foods. In addition, a great deal of water and minerals (sodium, chloride and potassium) are lost in the watery portion of the diarrheal stool; if you are not careful this can lead to dehydration. Patients with diarrhea have to drink considerably more fluid than usual to prevent the dehydration. This is especially important if the patient also has a fever, which in itself leads to increased loss of body water through the skin as perspiration.

In most cases, patients with diarrhea can tolerate a clear liquid diet without cramping or diarrhea. This is because the small intestine can absorb water, minerals and sugars pretty well even when infected. As the name implies, the diet starts off with clear liquids only. As symptoms abate, the diet slowly adds simple-to-digest, low-residue foods, one step at a time. Don't advance to the next step until the patient is completely symptom-free in the present step. As the patient progresses through each step, if the cramps and diarrhea return, drop back to the previous step they tolerated.

This same Clear Liquid Diet approach is the one to use for patients who have been ill with the flu and have been too ill to eat. They will have been on Step 1 already so when they become hungry, begin them on Step 2 and advance them through the steps as above.

Step 1: Oral Rehydration Solution (ORS), water, fruit juice, Jell-O, Gatorade or PowerAid, ginger ale, Sprite, tea.

Step 2: Add white toast (no butter or margarine), white rice, and cream of wheat, soda crackers, and potatoes without the skin.

Step 3: To Steps 1 and 2, add canned fruit and chicken noodle soup.

Step 4: To Steps 1 through 3, add poached eggs and baked chicken breast without skin, canned fish or meat.[26]

Step 5: To Steps 1 through 4, add milk and other dairy products, margarine or butter, raw fruits and vegetables and high-fiber whole grain products.

By recognizing the symptoms a patient has or the signs of the disease in the body, you can use the chart below to guide your treatment. Here's how.

Symptom or Sign	Likely Assessment	Remedy[27]
Low urine output	Dehydration	Push fluids
High pulse rate (>80 but especially > 90)	Dehydration or fever	Push fluids
Shortness of breath	Pneumonia	Push fluids
Shaking, chills and shivers	Viremia (virus in the blood) or pneumonia	Keep warm
Cyanosis (skin turns blue)	Respiratory failure, death likely	Keep as comfortable as possible. Give hydrocodone with promethazine for comfort, give diazepam for anxiety
Bleeding from mouth, coughing up blood, passing red blood per rectum. Severe bruising.	A severe blood clotting abnormality has occurred due to the virus (DIC). Death is likely	Keep as comfortable as possible. Give hydrocodone with promethazine for comfort, give diazepam for anxiety
Vomiting	Virus affecting GI tract	Use promethazine for vomiting, push fluids

Symptom or Sign	Likely Assessment	Remedy[27]
Diarrhea	Virus affecting GI tract	Push fluids, clear liquid diet
Severe stomach cramps	Virus affecting GI tract	Use hydrocodone and promethazine for comfort
Headache		Ibuprofen and/or acetaminophen or hydrocodone if very severe
Fever		Ibuprofen, acetaminophen, push fluids, keep warm or cool, consider tepid water baths if > 102 F. OK if <101 as this may help kill virus.
Sore throat		Gargle with hot salt water; drink hot tea or hot water, ibuprofen and or acetaminophen.
Cough		Push fluids, drink hot tea for effect on breathing tubes, use hydrocodone 1/2 tablet with or without 1/2 promethazine to suppress cough if needed

Advanced Home Treatment for Health Professionals

If you have access to Tamiflu, the dose is one tablet twice daily for five days. It is best to begin Tamiflu within two days of the beginning of symptoms but might be useful when used even later in the course.

Tamiflu Re-Administration Strategy

Tamiflu is excreted unchanged almost entirely in the urine. If Tamiflu supplies are limited, as they most certainly will be, consider giving the patient two Tamiflu tablets at the same time, collect the patient's urine and re-administer it to the patient via naso-gastric (NG) tube or orally. If managed carefully, this approach means that you can completely treat a patient with only two Tamiflu tablets.

To replace fluids using this method, dilute the urine to a specific gravity (SG) of 1.010 with plain water to reduce the electrolyte concentration and raise the pH of the urine to 7.4 by addition crushed $CaCo3$ (Tums) tablets to the solution and add sugar for glucose calories. Cool and flavor with citrus to improve palatability and administer orally or by NG tube.

Consider using homemade NG tubes by adapting any source of small gage plastic tubing. Urine should be administered as a cool beverage and as fresh as possible to reduce odor and taste from urea breakdown. Urine is non-toxic. Most of the toxic things are metabolized by the liver and excreted in the bile. Don't worry about urea, it is readily reabsorbed by the body and excreted back into the urine over and over again. It is non-toxic and will all come out once the urine is no longer being re-administered to the patient.

Management of Dehydration Using Urine SG

Urine specific gravity is best measured using a hand held refractometer. You can also use a urine dipstick to estimate SG. Urine SG is an excellent objective measure of the state of patient's hydration given normal renal function. Urine SG ranges from 1.000 (distilled water) to 1.035 (really concentrated). Normal kidneys can easily concentrate urine to 1.020 or above without difficulty after a typical overnight fast. Patients with chronic renal insufficiency are not able to concentrate urine much above 1.010. A clinically dehydrated patient with a urine SG of 1.010 is diagnostic of renal failure.

Recommendation: Adjust the rate of oral fluid administration to maintain the urine SG between 1.010 and 1.020.

Above all, in spite of the challenges and the disappointments, realize that you are doing the best you can.

Citizen Advocacy:
Helping Others Prepare

In addition to getting ready to handle whatever situation comes along for yourself and your family, I urge you to be active as a citizen. Since I began to write what became this manual, back in May 2005, there has been an explosion of interest and concern about a pandemic. Some national, state and local authorities are beginning to see that getting ready to face the risk of a pandemic is necessary.

As I write this, news reports say the long-delayed final version of the U.S. Pandemic Influenza Preparedness and Response Plan will soon be released. Adding your voice can make it more probable that enough is done, soon enough, if nature is kind and the pandemic is delayed. By all means communicate with your elected officials at the national level in favor of funding for vaccine and antiviral research, production, and stockpiling. Mention that providing substantial targeted aid to help find and contain outbreaks of avian flu in Asian countries is in our own country's interest as well.

If the pandemic arrives in the winter of 2005/6, as I fear it might, or even within the next couple of years, there is no realistic prospect of being "ready" in a medical sense with enough vaccines and antiviral drugs for everyone at risk. But this does NOT mean there is nothing that can be done now to reduce the pandemic's impact. Has your locality made realistic plans for dealing with a major pandemic? And have these contingency plans been practiced, either in dress rehearsals or "tabletop exercises," giving people who would need to coordinate during the actual emergency a chance to get to know each other?

If and when a pandemic starts, reducing person-to-person contact in school, work and other public settings would slow down the spread of the virus. How this would be arranged needs to be thought about now. As has already been discussed, the degree of absenteeism that would result from a major pandemic would interfere with the delivery of all sorts of essential goods and services, and puts the continuation of electricity, natural gas, and water supplies at risk. Have your local public utilities planned for 30 percent of their workforce not showing up (whether due to their own illness, taking care of family members, or just concern about getting infected)? Do they have enough of their essential raw materials, fuel, etc. in stock to go on for two or three months when rail and truck service might be spotty at best?

Now that you've read this manual, you know much more about the situation we face than most of your neighbors. If you believe what you've read here, you want to spread the news. Yes, of course—just as I'm doing now by writing this. But recognize that not everyone will want to hear it. Some of your family and friends will reject this information and call you a "Chicken Little" for being concerned and making preparations. They will rely upon the reassuring statements made by over-optimistic officials and "experts," or think that our relative prosperity will protect us. Others, however, may be open to learning and doing more. In sharing this information with them, make allowances for the fact that it is frightening. It's natural to have an "adjustment reaction" upon learning about this. Make it clear that there are things they can do for themselves and their family, and that though they may have sleepless nights they can expect to adjust to the "new normal."

Maybe the pandemic won't come for years, and when it does it could be relatively mild. But that is something we can't know now. Does a school that has fire drills waste the time of the teachers and students? No, it doesn't, even if there is never a fire. In the same way, you have not wasted your efforts if you prepare for a pandemic even if it doesn't come in your lifetime—because it might, and you will want to be ready if it does.

A Doctor's Letter During the Spanish Flu[28]

In September 1918, the second pandemic influenza wave was making its way through the America. Military bases were especially hard hit by the pandemic in the US. Below is a reprint of a letter found in 1959 in a trunk among other papers given to the Department of Epidemiology of the University of Michigan. Dr. N. R. Grist wrote this letter, published in the *British Medical Journal* in the December 22, 1979 issue as part of an article on the 1918 pandemic. Roy Grist was a recently recruited military doctor assigned to a US Army base in Massachusetts, Camp Devens. This was a training base for new recruits and was one of the worst affected by the flu. The letter is important for its clear description of the rapid course of the illness, how this pandemic flu differed so greatly from the usual seasonal variety, and how the medical resources of the camp had become exhausted by the sheer number of cases and the high case fatality rate.

Camp Devens, Mass.
Surgical Ward No 16
29 September 1918
(Base Hospital)

My dear Burt—

It is more than likely that you would be interested in the news of this place, for there is a possibility that you will be assigned here for duty, so having a minute between rounds I will try to tell you a little about the situation here as I have seen it in the last week.

As you know I have not seen much Pneumonia in the last few years in Detroit, so when I came here I was some- what behind in the niceties of the Army way of intricate Diagnosis. Also to make it good, I have had for the last week an exacerbation of my old "Ear Rot" as Artie Ogle calls it, and could not use a Stethoscope at all, but had to get by on my ability to "spot" ' em thru my general knowl- edge of Pneumonias. I did well enough, and finally found an old Phonendoscope that I pieced together, and from then on was all right. You know the Army regulations require very close locations etc.

Camp Devens is near Boston, and has about 50,000 men, or did have before this epidemic broke loose. It also has the Base Hospital for the Div. of the N. East. This epidemic started about four weeks ago, and has developed so rapidly that the camp is demoralized and all ordinary work is held up till it has passed. All assemblages of soldiers taboo.

These men start with what appears to be an ordinary attack of LaGrippe or Influenza, and when brought to the Hosp. they very rapidly develop the most vicious type of Pneumonia that has ever been seen. Two hours after admission they have the Mahogany spots over the cheek bones, and a few hours later you can begin to see the Cyanosis extending from their ears and spreading all over the face, until it is hard to distinguish the colored men from the white. It is only a matter of a few hours then until death comes, and it is simply a struggle for air until they suffocate. It is horrible. One can stand it to see one, two or twenty men die, but to see these poor devils dropping like flies sort of gets on your nerves. We have been averaging about 100 deaths per day, and still keeping it up. There is no doubt in my mind that there is a new mixed infection here, but what I dont know. My total time is taken up hunting Rales, rales dry or moist, sibilant or crepitant or any other of the hundred things that one may find in the chest, they all mean but one thing here—Pneumonia—

and that means in about all cases death.

The normal number of resident Drs. here is about 25 and that has been increased to over 250, all of whom (of course excepting me) have temporary orders—"Return to your proper Station on completion of work". Mine says "Permanent Duty", but I have been in the Army just long enough to learn that it doesn't always mean what it says. So I dont know what will happen to me at the end of this.

We have lost an outrageous number of Nurses and Drs., and the little town of Ayer is a sight. It takes Special trains to carry away the dead. For several days there were no coffins and the bodies piled up something fierce, we used to go down to the morgue (which is just back of my ward) and look at the boys laid out in long rows. It beats any sight they ever had in France after a battle. An extra long barracks has been vacated for the use of the Morgue, and it would make any man sit up and take notice to walk down the long lines of dead soldiers all dressed and laid out in double rows. We have no relief here, you get up in the morning at 5:30 and work steady till about 9.30 P.M., sleep, then go at it again. Some of the men of course have been here all the time, and they are TIRED.

If this letter seems somewhat disconnected overlook it,

for I have been called away from it a dozen times the last time just now by the Officer of the Day, who came in to tell me that they have not as yet found at any of the autopsies any case beyond the red hepatitis stage. It kills them before they get that far.

I don't wish you any hard luck Old Man but I do wish you were here for a while at least. It's more comfortable when one has a friend about. The men here are all good fellows, but I get so damned sick of Pneumonia that when I go to eat I want to find some fellow who will not "Talk Shop" but there ain't none nohow. We eat it, live it, sleep it, and dream it, to say nothing of breathing it 16 hours a day. I would be very grateful indeed if you would drop me a line or two once in a while, and I will promise you that if you ever get into a fix like this, I will do the same for you.

Each man here gets a ward with about 150 beds, (Mine has 168) and has an Asst. Chief to boss him, and you can imagine what the paper work alone is—fierce—and the Govt. demands all paper work be kept up in good shape. I have only four day nurses and five night nurses (female) a ward-master, and four orderlies. So you can see that we are busy. I write this in piecemeal fashion. It may be a long time before I can get another letter to you, but will try.

This letter will give you an idea of the monthly report, which has to be in Monday. I have mine most ready now. My Boss was in just now and gave me a lot more work to do so I will have to close this.

Good Bye old Pal,
"God be with you till we meet again"
Keep the Bowels open.
(Sgd) Roy.

How to Find Out More

Medical scientists around the world are closely monitoring the situation in Southeast Asia and regularly make reports that are published in the medical, scientific and lay press. You can follow these reports best using the Internet. To start, use the Google News service at *www.news.google.com* to search for articles relating to "avian influenza". This is one of the best ways to keep up-to-date on what is happening in Southeast Asia, which is the most likely place for the pandemic to begin.

One of the most informative sources of information is the historical account of the 1918 Spanish Flu written by John Barry entitled, *The Great Influenza*. This book is widely available in bookstores and on *www.amazon.com*. This excellent work chronicled the worldwide epidemic from start to finish and provided me with a new perspective on just how serious influenza can be when the conditions are right as they are today. What I found most interesting in Barry's book were the many first hand accounts of how the pandemic struck the U.S. and the world and just how devastating the illness was. The total inability of our institutions to stand up to the stress placed upon it by the 1918 pandemic was particularly enlightening for me.

I highly recommend you read about the 1918 flu pandemic since we could be on the verge of a similar event. Start by using Google to search for "1918 Spanish Flu". You will find a lot of information about that event. By learning more about the 1918 event, you will be able to fill in many of the details about this developing crisis we may be facing today. For those of you who remain in doubt about how serious a crisis this actually is, researching this issue on your own should help you develop a better appreciation of the situation.

Another book that does an excellent job of laying out the danger we face is *The Monster at Our Door: The Global Threat of Avian Flu*, by Mike Davis. He offers a valuable discussion of the biology of the influenza virus, and how the ecology of poultry and livestock living in close contact with people has promoted the development and spread of this potential pandemic.

Another wonderful book is *America's Forgotten Pandemic: The Influenza of 1918* by Alfred W. Crosby.

While putting this manual together, I discovered several very informative web sites that you will want to visit on a regular basis to keep up with pandemic developments. The first is *www.recombinomics.com*, a site maintained and authored by Henry L. Niman, Ph.D., a virologist with a special interest in recombinant viruses like influenza. He provides an excellent commentary on avian influenza events worldwide and usually has information on new developments and his commentary on their significance before virtually any other site.

The second is *www.fluwikie.com*. This site is dedicated to the avian flu pandemic and all aspects of it. It is a one-stop shop for anyone interested in the topic. It also has bulletin board with an active online community, and a list of other recommended links for keeping up with the news on this issue.

Finally, *Nature,* the international journal of science, has an avian influenza web page that has a collection of staff-written articles on the developing pandemic over the last few years. This is a wonderful resource for anyone interested in learning more about past as well as future pandemic developments: *www.nature.com/ nature/focus/avianflu.*

Approximate Spread of the 1918 Pandemic Across the U.S.

Approximate beginning of the epidemic, 1918

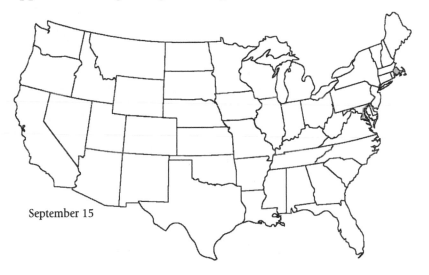

September 15

The following maps show the spread of the second, most deadly wave of the 1918 Spanish Flu pandemic

Dark areas represent areas of infection.

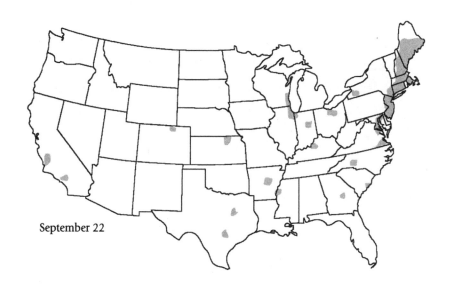

September 22

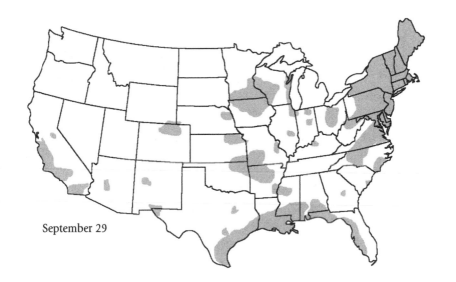

September 29

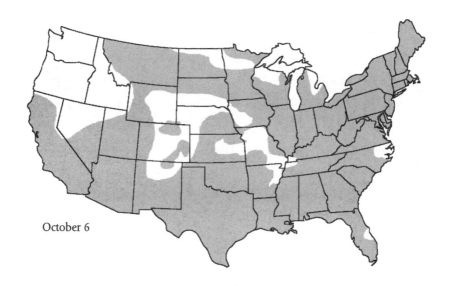

October 6

By the end of September, almost the entire country was affected by the pandemic.

Source: *America's Forgotten Pandemic: The Influenza of 1918*, Alfred W. Crosby, Cambridge University Press

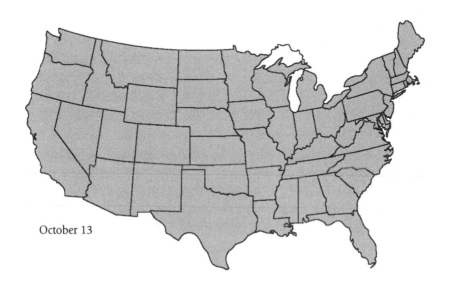

October 13

The pandemic reached its height in early October 1918 and then began to recede—but not before killing millions of people.

Endnotes

1 K. Ungchusak et al. Probable person-to-person transmission of acian influenza A (H5N1), N Engl J Med 2005; 352-333-40.

2 Director of the Center for Infectious Disease Research and Policy, the associate director of the National Center for Food Protection and Defense, and a professor of public health at the University of Minnesota, Minneapolis

3 M Osterholm, Preparing for the next pandemic, N Engl J Med 2005;352:1839-1842

4 Draft Pandemic Influenza Preparedness and Response Plan, DHHS, August 2004

5 UK Health Protection Agency Pandemic Plan for Influenza Feb 2005

6 Statement of Dominick A. Iacuzio, Ph.D., medical director, Hoffmann-La Roche, Inc, before the subcommittee on Health, Energy and Commence, United States House of Representatives, May 26, 2005.

7 H. Yen et al. Virulence may determine the necessary duration and dosage of Oselramivir treatment for highly pathogenic A/Vietnam/ 1203/04 (H5N1) influenza virus in mice. Journal of Infectious Diseases; 10.1086/432008 (2005)

8 Avian flu: Isolation of drug-resistant H5N1 virus, Q. Mai Le et al., Nature 437, 1108, October 20, 2005.

9 United Nations, World Urbanization Prospects, The 1999 Revision.

10 This prediction is based upon the time period when the next pandemic is most likely to begin. If we escape the pandemic during the 2005-06 flu seasons, unfortunately this does not get us off the hook. The pandemic risk simply rises until the event finally occurs since there is a 100 percent likelihood that it will happen. The advice given in this manual will be useful irrespective of when the flu pandemic strikes, especially if it is a major pandemic.

11 From the FEMA Web site: How to correctly boil or disinfect water. Hold water at a rolling boil for 1 minute to kill bacteria. If you can't boil water, add 1/8 teaspoon (~0.75 mL) of newly purchased, unscented liquid household bleach per gallon of water. Stir the water well, and let it stand for 30 minutes before you use it. You can use water-purifying tablets instead of boiling water or using bleach. For infants, use only pre-prepared canned baby formula. Do not use powdered formulas prepared with treated water. Clean children's toys that have come in contact with water. Use a solution of 1 cup of bleach in 5 gallons of water to clean the toys. Let toys air-dry after cleaning.

12 The US Federal Emergency Management Association recommends using household bleach to purify water for drinking by adding 1/8th tsp per gallon of water (1:7500 solution). To make a bleach disinfecting solution to contaminate surfaces and instruments mix 1-cup bleach to 1 gallon of water (1:10 solution). For general disinfectant purposes, the FEMA recommends 1-cup bleach to 5 gallons of water (1:50 solution).

13 Thermometers break so have more than one on hand.

14 I recommend the hand pumped automatic BP monitor rather than ones with electric pumps.

15 Tamiflu is expensive, costing about $200 for 20 tablets. If you have insurance, you will still pay stiff co-pay. All the other prescription drugs are generic and not expensive.

16 For the purposes of this guide, ibuprofen means aspirin, Advil, Aleve, ibuprofen, or Nuprin since they are all alike. Acetaminophen (Tylenol) is not an aspirin.

17 The ORS formula is excellent for treatment of dehydration due to all causes. If the patient has become dehydrated because of diarrhea, you can substitute the salt in the formula with 1/2 tsp of baking soda (if available) because diarrhea leads to loss of alkali.

18 Don't use more salt or baking soda in the ORS formula. I am already recommending the maximum dose of these.

19 The Writing Committee of the World Health Organization (WHO) Consultation on Human Influenza A/H5, N Engl J Med 2005; 353:1374-1385

20 The SOAP medical note format is a useful way to record medical information on patients. "S" is for subjective and used for what the patient tells you about their illness. This includes how they feel, what hurts and where, what they did for the symptoms, etc. "O" stands for objective and includes the things you observed or measured. This means her vital signs, skin tone, fluid in and urine out. "A" is your assessment of the patient's medical condition. "P" is the plan you make for helping the patient get better. I use this method in my practice and suggest it to you for your patient notes too.

21 Temperature can be measured in degrees F or C which ever is most

familiar to you. In this manual, I use degrees in F.

22 The pulse is usually regular, like a tom-tom drum. The beats are equally spaced and occur regularly. If you tap your toe to the pulse, a regular pulse is one that occurs predictably one beat after another. A regular pulse is normal. An irregular pulse is not. Having an occasional extra beat or drop beat is OK. A very fast irregular pulse can be a problem. This gets too complicated for me to give you specific advice except to say that a regular fast pulse in the context of flu suggests dehydration is present.

23 Normal respiratory rates are in the range of 12 to 16 breaths per minute. Fever and dehydration are associated with faster respiratory rates. Acidosis from massive infection is also a cause of high respiratory rates. When patients are near death, the respiratory rate slows down and becomes more and more shallow.

24 Normal BP is 120/80 or so but there is a wide range of normal from a low of 90/60 for teens and girls to 140/90 for some adults. Pressures below 90/60 are usually abnormal and in the context of flu due to dehydration. These low BPs are often associated with a high pulse. Try and keep the patient's BP above 100 on the top and 60 on the bottom if possible.

25 Fluid in and out is best measured in milliliters (ml). Most kitchen measuring cups are graduated in both ml and ounces/cups.

26 Sick patients break down their muscle tissue for needed protein and calories. This is fine as long as it does not go on for long. It is important to begin feeding the patient high quality animal protein as soon as they can tolerate it to help them maintain their strength.

27 Are these the right treatments for this symptom in every case? Of

course not! I am providing you with my best guess of how to manage the average very sick flu patient, but not every very sick flu patient. I recognize that for some like those with Acute Respiratory Distress Syndrome (ADRS) or congestive heart failure for instance, these suggestions will not be helpful and would be considered harmful under usual circumstances. You will not be able to tell when you are dealing with one of these rare patients. So, what should you do? For most patients, following the advice will do a lot of good and makes the most sense under these unique circumstances. All you can do is the best you can do. So do that with a satisfied mind. You can't save every patient. Don't let any tragic loss prevent you from keeping faith in your ability to help most patients with the techniques found here. You are their only hope.

28 Published in the British Medical Journal, December 22, 1979

About the Author

Grattan Woodson, M.D., FACP obtained his MD at the Medical College of Georgia in 1980 and completed his internal medicine training at an affiliate of Columbia University College of Physicians and Surgeons in New York, New York in 1983. He joined the full-time faculty of Emory University School of Medicine where he taught internal medicine and worked as a diagnostician at Emory Clinic. Presently he is an attending physician at the Druid Oaks Health Center in Decatur, Georgia.

Dr. Woodson first became concerned about avian influenza after learning about the first human cases in Hong Kong in 1997. His interest increased significantly when the disease re-emerged in Southeast Asia in 2003. As the disease has evolved it became evident to him that the likelihood of a worldwide influenza pandemic similar to the devastating 1918 Spanish Flu was increasing. In order to prepare his patients for a possible catastrophic event. Dr. Woodson has authored this manual.

About the Editor

D avid Jodrey, Ph.D., earned his doctorate in psychology at the State University of New York at Buffalo. He has taught there, in Virginia, and at Johns Hopkins University, where he was also a Research Associate at the School of Public Health. Recently he was certified in Hanna Somatic Education, an approach to overcoming pain and movement limitations (see *www.somatics.org*).

NOTES

Germ Freaks Unite!

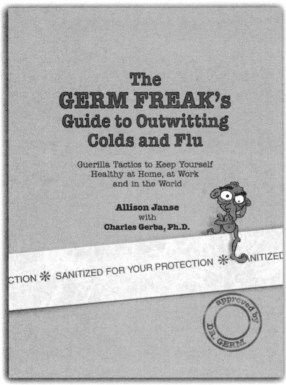

Code #3277 • $11.95

This light-hearted but eminently practical book combines the knowledge of one of the world's top infectious disease experts with real world tactics of an everyday germ freak. Together, they give you straight answers on staying healthy with your sanity intact.